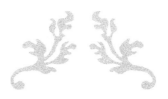

INTERMITTENT FASTING
FOR WOMEN

A complete guide to start eating well, regain confidence, reset
metabolism and lose weight to stay fit with easy and fast recipes

JOSEPHINE BERG

indirect, which are incurred as a result of the use of information contained within this document, including, but not limited to, — errors, omissions, or inaccuracies.

Table of Contents

Introduction.. 10

Chapter 1.   What Is Intermittent Fasting? 16

What Is Intermittent Fasting?... 16

How Does IF Work? 17

Why Does IF Works? 18

What Effects Does It Have on Your Body Hormones?............. 18

1. Fat Loss and Hunger Hormones: (Leptin, Insulin, + Ghrelin)
.... 19

2. Estrogen and Progesterone.. 20

3. Adrenal Hormones (Cortisol).. 20

4. Thyroid Hormones 21

Plan of Intermittent Fasting, If You Are:..................................... 21

Beginners.. 21

Intermediate... 22

Advanced 22

Chapter 2.   Methods of Intermittent Fasting 24

The 16/8 Method.. 24

The Importance of Your Circadian Rhythm............................... 26

The 5:2 Diet 27

Eat-Stop-Eat Diet 27

Alternate Day Fasting... 29

Warrior Diet... 29

Spontaneous Meal Skipping... 30

Extended Fasting.. 31

Chapter 3.   Balancing Hormones and Increasing Energy 33

Hormones..34

Energy..37

Chapter 4.   Myths about Intermittent Fasting 42

Fasting Is Dangerous...42

Fasting Can Lower Your Blood Sugar Dangerously....................42

It Will Cause Hormonal Imbalance...................................43

It Will Destroy Your Metabolism....................................43

It Causes Stress...44

Fasting Can Lead to Overeating.....................................45

Fasting Causes the Body to Go into Starvation Mode.................45

Fasting Causes the Body to Burn Muscle.............................45

You Can't Work Out While Fasting...................................46

Chapter 5.   Metabolic Effects of Fasting.......................48

Therapeutic (intermittent) Fasting.................................51

Therapeutic Fasting..52

Fasting According to Alternative Medicine..........................54

Chapter 6.   Foods and Drinks Suitable for Intermittent Fasting 57

Chapter 7.   Activating Autophagy................................65

What Is Autophagy and How Does It Work? 65

The Science Behind Autophagy.......................................67

The Benefits 68

How to Activate Autophagy..70

Chapter 8.   Ideal Diet in Menopause.............................73

What Happens to the Body of a Menopausal Woman?....................73

The Ideal Diet for Menopause.......................................75

Chapter 9.   Is Intermittent Fasting Safe for Older Adults?......79

What to Consider Before You Start Your Journey to Weight Loss 80

5 Tips for Intermittent Fasting Everyone Should Know 81

Prepare to Your Fast 81

Use Supplements to Make Your Fasting Days Better 82

It Might Not Be Any More 82

On Fasting Days, Drink More Tea 82

Make Fasting Days More Like Days of Rest 82

Common Mistakes to Avoid During Intermittent Fasting 83

Mistake 1: You Can Only Drink Water in the Fasted State 83

Mistake 2: Being Overly Ambitious with Fasting 83

Mistake 3: The Longer Your Fast, the Better 83

Mistake 4: The Feeling of Hunger Is Bad for You 84

Mistake 5: Intermittent Fasting Is Not Good for Our Health 84

Mistake 6: Not Taking Enough Minerals 85

Mistake 7: Consuming Branched Chain Amino Acids 85

Mistake 8: Not Exercising 85

Sample Daily Plan for Intermittent Fasting 86

Chapter 10.   The Right Mindset When Starting IF 89

The Difference Between Needing and Wanting to Eat 89

There Is a Huge Difference Here 89

Eat Only When Needed 89

Hydration Is Essential 90

Take Things Slowly 90

Cut Down on Carbs and Sugar Even on Non-Fast Days 91

Keep Track of Your Achievements 92

Introduction

Fasting has been practiced in many different faith traditions since ancient times. The first recorded Christian practice of abstaining from food was done by Jesus Christ during his forty days in the desert. Although the Bible does not expressly mention fasting as a specific practice, it does recognize that people fasted for other religious purposes. The Hebrew word for fasting is "mazzah" which means to be hungry. All three of these practices are beneficial and healthful, however, the developing age of most modern-day women often makes fasting extremely difficult.

Fasting has been practiced by women for health reasons as well as when they feel God is calling upon them to fast during a time of mourning or repentance. However, many women have concerns about starting a practice such as intermittent fasting because they are afraid it will lead to malnutrition or even starvation. While there is some merit to this concern, it is not necessarily a negative outcome.

The history of fasting in the Christian faith dates back to the early part of the fourth century. The first known comprehensive work regarding fasting was a book written by Eusebius of Caesarea entitled "Praecellens Divinorum Officiorum Liber" (The Book of Divine Offices). Eusebius was a Roman historian who studied Greek and became a bishop after Emperor Constantine's conversion to Christianity. He also headed the Church at Jerusalem for some time before returning to Caesarea in Palestine, where he wrote this book in 303 AD. This book contains an entire chapter on the topic of fasting, in which Eusebius describes the different types of fasting, including the one we know as "partial fasting" which is more commonly referred to as "intermittent fasting," and was practiced by Christians.

There are two forms of intermittent fasting that are recognized by medical health experts today. The first form is called "periodical intermittent fasting" (or 16:8 for short) and includes fasting for at least 16 hours a day, sometimes as long as 24 hours. This type of intermittent fasting is typically used for weight loss and has been proven effective in reducing appetite and burning fat.

The second type of intermittent fasting is known as the "alternate day" fast and involves skipping a meal per day. This type of fasting is beneficial for people who have trouble sticking with one consistent fasting day because it allows for greater flexibility.

"Alternative fasting", also known as "intermittent fasting", refers to eating every other day and fasting every other day (no food or calorie drinks), usually once a week. It is called intermittent because the exact number of hours in between meals varies from person to person, but eating no food for at least 12 hours is recommended by some nutritionists. Although it may be difficult to stick with fasting for 16 hours a day, intermittent fasting can be very effective if done correctly. It will help you lose weight, feel more energetic, and prevent or heal many diseases.

So why is intermittent fasting beneficial? Most importantly, it helps to lose weight. In a study, published in Cell Metabolism, it was shown that intermittent fasting caused an average of 3-7% decreases in body fat and increases in muscle mass for obese mice. It also increased their lifespan by 36%. The researchers concluded that the benefit of a healthy diet can be extended by periodic fasting.

Fasting is also known to improve your health and prevent or reverse heart disease and cancer as well as many other diseases. In a study conducted at UCLA, it was discovered that aspirin increases the life span in mice when combined with fasting or caloric restriction.

In addition to proven benefits, intermittent fasting has also been shown to reduce caloric intake and encourage the individual to focus on healthier meals. It is particularly useful for people who are overweight but do not have time to focus on every meal of the day, as well as people who have difficulty controlling their appetite. It is an excellent way to lose weight while improving health and quality of life. There are several ways to practice intermittent fasting, all of which will help you lose weight.

Intermittent fasting is "alternating day" fasting, it involves eating normally for 24 hours and then not eating anything, either on a day when you're free or on Friday, the day that Christians traditionally do not eat meat. After this 24-hour period of abstinence from food, one can eat as much as desired on that day. However, the individual must only eat within a 12-hour window. This means that you should not eat your first meal until 12 hours have passed since your last meal and then follow with a second meal twelve hours after that.

Another form of intermittent fasting, known as time-restricted feeding, is where the person restricts his eating to within a certain period. For instance, one could eat breakfast at 9:00 a.m. and then not eat anything again until 10:00 a.m., lunch at noon, and then not eat anything again until 1:00 p.m., and so on.

Whichever form you choose to implement in your life, make sure that you keep track of what you're eating on a particular day, and do not deviate from this schedule. This will help you to adjust your pattern of eating if necessary when new foods are introduced or if you feel that it may be leading to overeating. It will also help you to keep up with your regular schedule and avoid falling out of the habit.

Although intermittent fasting can be effective, it is still an approach that requires some practice. You must decide if it will be a daily or weekly practice for you, depending on your lifestyle and how much time is available. If you have a lot of time available and are dedicated to following this type of eating plan for the long-term, then intermittent fasting may be a good plan for you.

Chapter 1. What Is Intermittent Fasting?

It isn't an eating routine, it's a way of eating. It's a method for booking your dinners so you benefit from them. It doesn't change what you eat, it changes when you eat. This is an unconventional way to lose weight without having to eat crazy or reduce calories to zero. Indeed, more often than not you'll attempt to keep your calories a similar when you start discontinuous fasting. (The vast majority eat greater suppers during a shorter time allotment.) Additionally, it is a decent method to keep bulk on while getting lean. With all that stated, the major reason individuals attempt this kind of fasting is to lose fat. Maybe, in particular, irregular fasting is perhaps the least complex procedure we have for losing weight in light of the fact that it requires almost no behavior change. This is an excellent advantage. Since it implies discontinuous fasting, it falls into the class of "basic enough that you'll really do it, however significant enough that it will really have any kind of effect."

To see how IF prompts fat loss, we first need to understand the distinction between the fed state and the fasted state. Your body is in the fed state when it is processing and retaining nourishment. Regularly, the fed state begins when you start eating and goes on for three to five hours as your body processes and retains the nourishment you just ate. When you are in the fed express, it's exceptionally difficult for your body to consume fat because your insulin levels are high. After that period, your body goes into what is known as the post-absorptive state, which is only an extravagant method for saying that your body isn't handling a feast. The post-absorptive state goes on until 8 to 12 hours after your last supper, which is the point at which you enter the fasted state. It is a lot simpler for your body to consume fat in the fasted state in light of the fact that your insulin levels are low. When you're in the fasted state—some 12 hours after our last supper—your body can consume fat that has been out of reach during the fed period. Since we don't enter the fasted state until, it's uncommon that our bodies are right now state. This is one reason why numerous individuals who start intermittent fasting will lose fat without changing what they eat, the amount they eat, or how regularly they work out. Fasting places your body in a fat-consuming state that you once in a while make it happen during a typical eating plan.

Why Does IF Works?

While IF might be a mainstream pattern in the eating regimen world nowadays, those attempting to get thinner or improve their general wellbeing should realize that it tends to be a hard arrangement to stick to. The methodology shifts back and forth between times of fasting and non-fasting during a specific timeframe. IF isn't about hardship, however, about separating your calories uniquely in contrast to the three-full dinners daily in addition to a nibble routine. The explanation IF is believed to be successful in weight reduction is on the grounds that it expands your body's responsiveness to insulin. Insulin, a hormone that is discharged when you eat, causes your liver, muscle, and fat cells to store glucose. In a fasting state, blood glucose levels drop, which prompts a dropping in insulin creation, flagging your body to begin consuming energy. Following 12 hours of fasting, your body comes up short on reserve energy and starts consuming fat stores to generate it.

What Effects Does It Have on Your Body Hormones?

The advantages of IF are buzzing in the wellbeing scene with inquiries about supporting its capacity to decrease inflammation, heal the gut, and increment cell repair. While restricting nourishment admission for a while can do to ponder for your wellbeing, there are a few concerns in regards to the potential symptoms it could have on hormonal wellbeing, particularly for those with thyroid issues, adrenal weakness, or other hormone uneven characters. So how about we jump profoundly into the hormone-fasting association with assistance and decide whether this could be a decent mending device for you:

1. Fat Loss and Hunger Hormones: (Leptin, Insulin, + Ghrelin)

Intermittent fasting becomes the overwhelming focus in its job in improving yearning, digestion, and glucose influencing hormones. When patients come in with blood sugar problems, it's good to prescribe IF because of its demonstrated capacity to increase metabolism and lower insulin obstruction. If you have a glucose issue and need to have a go at fasting, it's vital to work with your primary care physician who can screen you and increment your length of fasting as your glucose stabilizes. Leptin opposition, another hormonal obstruction design that prompts weight gains and weight reduction, has likewise been demonstrated to improve with IF.

What's more, if you figure fasting would make you increasingly eager, reconsider. Intermittent fasting has been appeared to emphatically influence the craving hormone ghrelin, which can directly improve brain dopamine levels. This is the ideal case of the truth of the gut-mind pivot association.

2. Estrogen and Progesterone

Your brain and ovaries are connected through the ovary hub or hypothalamic-pituitary-gonadal (HPG) axis. Your cerebrum discharges hormones to your ovaries to flag them to discharge estrogen and progesterone. If your HPG hub isn't functioning correctly, it can influence your general health. With regards to IF, ladies are generally more delicate than men. This is because of the way that ladies have more loss of leptin, which makes more noteworthy affectability to fasting. If not done appropriately, IF can make ladies mess up their cycle and lose their hormones. While more research should be done, it would bode well to legitimately reason that this hormonal move could influence digestion and health as well.

Presently this to state, since each individual is unique, this doesn't mean you can never attempt intermittent fasting. You may simply need to go at it with an alternate methodology. This can be an incredible method to systematically bring fasting into your daily schedule.

3. Adrenal Hormones (Cortisol)

Cortisol is your body's fundamental pressure hormone and is discharged by your adrenal organs which sit directly on your kidneys. When your mind adrenal (HPA) hub is lost, it can prompt problems in cortisol. This high and low rollercoaster winds up driving to adrenal weakness. I've discovered that individuals with dysfunctions with their circadian beat don't deal with intermittent fasting very well. Nonetheless, attempting a moderate novice intermittent fasting convention or crescendo fasting could approve of somebody checking your advancement.

4. Thyroid Hormones

Your thyroid is sovereign of all hormones influencing every cell in your body. No other hormone has that power. There is a wide range of types of thyroid problems, all of which can be affected diversely by irregular fasting. Along these lines, it's good working with a useful medication professional who can work with your particular wellbeing case.

Plan of Intermittent Fasting, If You Are:

Beginners

The 8-6 window plan: One simple way to IF is to just eat between 8 am and 6 pm. This allows for a long fasting period within a reasonable timeframe.

The 12-6 window plan: I personally do this plan during my workweek. This is the same as the last plan but extends the fast a couple more hours into lunchtime. I fill my morning with big cups of water and antioxidant-rich matcha tea.

Modified 2-day plan: Eat clean for five days and then restrict calorie intake to 700 on any two other days. Limited calorie intake can have similar effects as full fasting.

The 5-2 plan: Eat clean for five days and fully fast for two nonconsecutive days a week.

Every-other-day plan: Fast fully every other day. While intense, it can be very effective for some people.

Chapter 2.

Chapter 2. Methods of Intermittent Fasting

The 16/8 Method

During this method, you have to fast for about 14 to 16 hours each day and eat the rest of the hours. During this feeding time, you can still take in two to three meals with no problem. This is more likely to fit in with the lunch schedule that you're used to, but it still affects you so you don't eat all day.

This approach is simpler than you'd expect. After dinner, it's as easy as not eating meals and then skipping breakfast or at least having a late snack. Okay, you're just fasting for 16 hours because you're finishing your last meal at 8 o'clock in the night and then eating nothing until midday the next day. Just be careful of the late-night therapies. Eating them in the morning will require you to skip the coffee.

Many people have issues with this because in the morning they feel hungry for food and they know they need to sleep. Only shift the meal to a bit later in the day. If you choose, for example, to eat breakfast at 10 a.m. You would still be within the 16-hour period instead of eight and then stop eating at 6 a.m.

As a woman, this form of intermittent fasting is advisable. With these shorter fasts, women typically do well and it is best to go fasting for 14 to 15 hours as this is more helpful to you.

During the fast, you are allowed to drink beer, tea, coffee, and other non-caloric liquids to help lessen hunger pains. In fact, you should try to stick to healthier foods during your feeding time. Eating a lot of unsanitary food during this time isn't a good idea. Many people like to have a low-carb diet when they are on an intermittent fast because it deals with fatigue and gives better outcomes.

The rationale behind the approach of 16/8 focuses on your hormonal rhythms and biological clock. According to Satchidananda Panda, a professor at the Salk Institute for Biological Studies and an expert in the field of biology and circadian rhythms, the body has not only one biological clock but several, which make up the full circadian rhythm. There's one biological clock in your liver, one in your kidneys, and one in your stomach, and according to Panda, each of these clocks was switched on and turned off at various times.

Shortly after you feed, the digestive system kicks in gear. When food moves through your digestive tract, every organ involved in the digestive process turns on, eats the food, and then turns off. When all digestive organs are shut off, it will allow the digestive system time to rest. During this time, the digestive system does its own "cleanup"— similar to a concept of a self-cleaning oven. Any remaining food residues are cleaned out, and the body is ready to start over again.

And if you constantly put food in your mouth, it will never shut down your digestive system, so it will never have enough time to perform its self-cleaning, which will have a negative impact on both your metabolism and overall health. Through his study, Panda found that giving the body an eight to twelve-hour, no-food window is best for your health. He claims it will help you lose weight (or maintain a healthy weight) and help stave off diabetes, high cholesterol, and obesity by introducing a daily fasting period.

The Importance of Your Circadian Rhythm

For fully understanding Panda's work, it is helpful to know what your circadian rhythm is, and how it affects the body. Also referred to as a body clock or biological clock, the circadian rhythm is a twenty-four-hour cycle that regulates many of the body's physiological processes, including sleep and digestion. The body gets signals from your circadian rhythm about when to go to sleep, when to wake up and when to feed.

Your circadian rhythm is regulated centrally by a brain area called the hypothalamus but is primarily influenced by natural environmental signals, such as temperature and light. For example, when it's dark outside, your eyes send a signal to your hypothalamus that it's time for you to sleep; your hypothalamus sends a message to the pineal gland (in another area of your brain) that activates melatonin (a hormone that helps you sleep), and you get sleepy. When it is light-out the opposite happens. Your eyes send your hypothalamus a signal, which tells your pineal gland to reduce the production of melatonin. A dip in melatonin will make you stand up and get ready for the day.

The 5:2 Diet

The 5:2 diet is another viable option. This fast advises you to eat normally for five days during the week and to limit yourself for each of the other two days to no more than 600 calories. This is sometimes called the Easy Diet, too.

It's recommended that on these fasting days, people will eat around 500 calories. You'll normally eat every day of the week, for example, and on Monday and Thursdays you'll have only two small meals with at least 500 calories. You can choose any day of the week as your fasting days, as long as you don't have them back to back. Choose your two busy days of the week and make them fasting days.

There aren't many reports out there about the 5:2 diet, but it will provide most of the benefits you're finding as it's intermittent fast. You can do it without the need to think all day about making meals.

Eat-Stop-Eat Diet

The Eat-Stop-Eat diet helps you skip 24-hour meals once or twice a week. This method was first popularized by Brad Pilon and has been a popular way to do the Intermittent Fasting for some time. You can do this fasting while still having one meal a day. Some citizens will have dinner every day and then eat nothing until the supper of the next day. It lets you never go a whole day without eating but still falling in the 24-hour abstinence process.

You do need to change that though. You can choose one of those options when going from breakfast to breakfast or lunch to lunch is best for you. During your fast, you are allowed to have coffee, water, and other non-caloric drinks to keep you hydrated, but you are not permitted to have any food at all.

Note that you're just fasting for one or two days a week. If it's time to eat properly, you need to consume the same amount of food you would have if you weren't on a fast. This will help you lose weight without hurting your body.

The only problem with getting on with this kind of Intermittent Fasting is that keeping it for 24 hours is hard for most people. Nonetheless, you can ease that. You can find that beginning with a shorter option, like the 16-hour fast, can produce some good results, and then continue to run for longer periods of time. Without food, it can be hard to go through a whole day and most people tend to go with one of the other fasting options to see the same effects.

Alternate Day Fasting

With this choice, the alternate day, you can take with you a few things, and it depends on what applies to your needs. Some of those fasts would allow you to have around 500 calories on your fasting days. Most sporadic laboratory studies used some version of the simple alternate day to help determine health benefits. Fasting every other day can be daunting to most people too!!!

It's certainly something you'll need to build up to every other day. It can be a struggle to push yourself to eat on alternate days. You'll probably feel very hungry many days a week on this fasting schedule, and it's hard to stick to that over the long run.

Warrior Diet

The warrior's way of fasting is remaining hungry for the entire day and then eating food at night. This can work well for people who are workaholics and do not have time to eat. This can also be very useful for people who are traveling far. Eating in a journey can be difficult and unwanted for a few people. If you train your body for the warrior diet, then you can easily skip eating during a long journey.

You can however have small portions of fruits and vegetables that are healthy during the day. Do not eat anything heavy though. For the warrior method of fasting, you get a 4 hours window to eat anything during the night.

Since it is called the warrior diet, you also should eat like how our warriors of ancient times used to eat, "unprocessed food". You should only eat foods that are not processed; basically "whole food" is the way to go with this method. Warrior fasting method is quite similar to the food choices we have in the "paleo diet".

Spontaneous Meal Skipping

You should do this if you want to prep your body for intermittent fasting, or if you don't want to spend a lot of time worrying about when you can drink. With this easy, you don't need to worry about following one of the more organized, intermittent fasting programs. You'll probably miss any meals occasionally. If you are not thirsty, or if you are too exhausted for a meal, you can do this. It is a big myth that you have to eat food every few hours to stop hunger.

The liver is well adapted without food, to last long periods. Waiting on a few meals isn't harmful to your health, particularly if you're not hungry or too busy.

If you end up eating a meal or two, you are actually fasting. If you are too busy to get a snack out of the door, just make sure you eat a good lunch and dinner. When you run out of errands and can't find a place to eat, then it's great to miss out on a snack. It will do no good and will really save you money.

You probably won't see results as good as some of the other options, but it's better than nothing and it's much easier to work with. Perhaps try skipping one or two meals during the week, or missing any meals when it's going for you.

As you can see, there are several different options you can deal with when you're ready to go on the Intermittent Fasting. You'll need to choose which pace to work in your everyday life is best.

Extended Fasting

Although extended fasting belongs to one class of its own, it is important to understand the difference between it and the other types of intermittent fasting. Extended fasting is any form of fast that lasts longer than 24 hours. Long fasting can often last for a week and many of these long fasts simply require drinking liquids.

These types of fasts are more normal throughout the medical and surgical settings and are usually done when the body needs to experience substantial recovery or when the ability to feed is impaired. Without the guidance and monitoring of a medical professional, you should not pursue this type of fasting.

Chapter 3. Balancing Hormones and Increasing Energy

Hormones are potent chemicals that convey messages through the body to manage specific processes. They are needed for growth, fertility, metabolism, and mood or behavior.

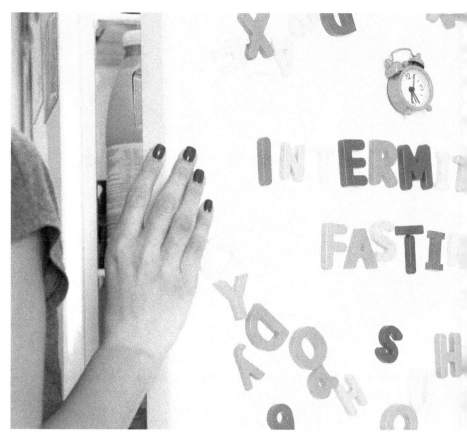

Hormones

As we age, our hormones change, and our body produces more of some, less of others. Hormones are made following the person's stage of life. For instance, a teenager's hormones are produced to urge them through puberty—the subsequent stage of development for the physical body where hair starts to develop in strategic places. A woman's body changes and starts to urge ready for the next step to supply offspring.

In pregnancy, the body produces the human chorionic gonadotropin (HCG) hormone. Also, as human placental lactogen (HPL) hormone, estrogen, and progesterone. As most people know, women seem to be everywhere both physically and emotionally once they expect. Now you recognize why these extremely potent chemicals are being produced.

Women undergo perimenopause, usually in their mid-forties. At this stage, the body's estrogen production starts to hamper until they are going through menopause. In menopause, the body stops releasing eggs, which suggests a lady is not any longer ready to reproduce.

Most women will undergo menopause between the ages of fifty-one to fifty-two. It can last anywhere from one to 3 years and the symptoms can include:

- The cycle has stopped for a year or more.

- Problems in sleeping.

- Bad nightly sweats, which will drench the person.

- Uncomfortably dry or itchy skin that seems like you've got a thousand ants crawling on you.

- Problems with urination, like releasing little drops when sneezing, problems urinating, and incontinence issues.

- Infections in the urinary tract or dryness, with a burning sensation

- A decreased libido and disinterest in intimacy

- Some women experience varying degrees of lethargy.

- Hot flashes that cause an individual to desire the doors of hell have opened ahead of them. These come on suddenly with no warning at any time or place in the day.

Some women will experience all of those symptoms. A number of them may get them more mildly or not in the least. Menopause and its symptoms resemble being pregnant. The hormones, or lack thereof, affect each woman differently. It wholly depends on how your body adjusts to the present, introduces its lifecycle.

It is vital to undertake and balance your hormones. One hormone which increases when practicing intermittent fasting is somatotropin. As soon as an individual stops eating for long enough, the body starts to supply this hormone. The hormone sent repairs tissue and is usually called the fountain of youth hormone thanks to its reparative qualities. While it doesn't do much to vary menopause, it'll help hamper the aging process and assist you in retaining muscle. It also helps with weight loss, and intermittent fasting has been shown to almost double this hormone in the body.

In menopause, two hormones that become imbalanced are melatonin and cortisol. These are the hormones that take to be in sync, as melatonin helps an individual sleep and luxuriate in good quality sleep. While cortisol is that hormone that allows an individual to awaken, feel alert, and keep the mind clear. An imbalance of those two hormones is typically thanks to ill health, anxiety, stress, and menopause. Intermittent fasting, alongside the right nutrition may aid in the production and balance of those two hormones.

Homeostasis is that the term used for hormone balance, and it's vital for optimum health. To achieve success with an intermittent fasting program, you furthermore may need a nutritious diet. Once a lady reaches fifty, it's imperative to measure a healthy lifestyle to make sure you enjoy your time of life in peak form.

Women over fifty should strive to:

- Eat well but healthy and make smarter food choices.

- Fast in their temperature and make it a neighborhood of their life.

- Take supplements to make sure they're getting enough vitamins and minerals.

- Take care of their skin by implementing the right treatments in or out of the sun.

- Wear protection in the heat when outside. Wear a hat to hide your face and neck. Wear sun protection, although an honest quarter-hour of direct sunlight will increase vitamin D.

- Exercise a minimum of two to 3 times every week, more if you're ready to.

- Most importantly, drink a lot of water.

Energy

Hormones can equally affect an individual's energy levels. In menstrual cycles, energy levels are known to spike and rise thanks to increased levels of estrogen. But after the process, the amount of estrogen drops quite drastically, causing lethargy. As women reach menopause and estrogen levels start to drop, women feel less energetic and very tired.

Another hormonal culprit that contributes to a menopausal woman's lack of energy is progesterone. This hormone declines with age and is one among the explanations middle-aged women have problems sleeping. Progesterone is employed to induce ovulation in younger ladies, but it also promotes sleep. A lady's browsing time of life does not need ovulation, so her body doesn't produce the maximum amount because it won't happen.

Although they do not produce it in the amounts a person does, an adult female body also has testosterone. Testosterone performs a big part in the production of red blood cells in the body. Red blood cells are the cells that transport oxygen around the body, which may be a much-needed component in the promotion of energy. Like many other hormones, menopause limits the production of testosterone also.

High-stress levels will cause a rise in cortisol, which, as discussed in the previous section, keeps an individual awake. This fact affects sleep patterns, which is merely another added factor causing a scarcity of energy thanks to feeling tired. It'll even have an impression on a woman's mood and leave them feeling horrible.

There are ways to extend energy levels, but the primary step to take is to rise your hormone levels. This fact will be done by your medical advisor, a registered clinic, or there are home tests you can acquire at the pharmacy. Ask a pharmacist what the most specific and most reliable brands are. Once you recognize what you're handling, there are a couple of methods you'll attempt to increase energy levels.

Never try hormone replacements or balancing hormones without the recommendation of a medical professional. If you're not on any medication or don't have any pre-existing medical conditions, you'll try one among the following tips:

- Ask your doctor, nutritionist, or pharmacist to recommend an honest quality multi-vitamin. Confirm you fall under a routine of taking them.

- Slowly change your diet to at least one that gives more nutrition and goes together with your system. As you age, you'll find foods that you simply may not be ready to eat.

- Find a quiet time to take ten to fifteen minutes to meditate, clear your mind, and learn the art of breathing.

- Tibetan monks have practiced anapanasati, which is mindfulness through breathing.

- Get enough good-quality sleep. You'll get to make some adjustments to your bedroom. Confirm your pillow is supporting your head, and your mattress is doing an equivalent for your body. Take all electronics out of your room; if you employ your mobile for an alarm, confirm it goes into sleep mode. Rather than a TV, make space for a chair to twist up in and skim. Reading before bed may be an excellent way to unwind and slip into another world to clear your mind. Try not to take naps during the day.

- Get in some exercise a minimum of once each day, twice if you'll manage it. It doesn't mean you've got to travel running a marathon or do the Tour de France. Choose a walk, do some gardening, or take a mild bike ride and appearance at the scenery.

- Find a replacement hobby or take up an old one you had forgotten. If you engage your mind, you'll automatically gear your body up for action.

- There are supplements and specific foods to boost your energy naturally. Whatever you are doing, don't try highly caffeinated drinks or other such sorts of energy boosters you discover in a supermarket.

By now, you know a subsequent little bit of advice goes to be — drink a lot of water. It's an excellent cure for an entire lot of things, including lethargy. If you would like to urge a touch extra boost, try using an icepack on your vagus in your neck for a moment at a time.

Chapter 4.

Chapter 4. Myths about Intermittent Fasting

There are so many myths about intermittent fasting circulating in health books and on the Internet. These erroneous statements have created a stigma around intermittent fasting that causes people to avoid following this breakthrough diet. Learn to see through these myths which are not true.

Fasting Is Dangerous

This first myth is simply ridiculous. Everyone intermittently fasts as they sleep. Doing it at other times or for a few days on end is no more dangerous than simply fasting while you sleep. The body needs a period to perform autophagy, and it cannot do that if it is too busy processing food all of the time. Intermittent fasting gives your body a well-deserved break while helping you preserve your health.

Remember, fasting is not starvation. You can still eat. Don't confuse fasting, which is healthful with starvation, which is dangerous.

Fasting Can Lower Your Blood Sugar Dangerously

The body can maintain its own blood glucose levels by releasing glycogen, or sugar stored in the liver. This fact means that you won't go low dangerously if you stop eating for a spell. Instead, it will balance out and cause your body to start burning fat. The fat will keep you nourished and prevent fainting from not eating.

If you feel faint or lightheaded, you may need to eat. Be sure to listen to your body. Decrease your fasting period if you keep having dizzy spells.

However, if you have diabetes or low blood sugar, you may need some help to maintain blood sugar levels during fasting. Ask your doctor how you can do this maintenance. Some fruit juice will technically break your fast, but it is necessary if your blood glucose plummets down.

It Will Cause Hormonal Imbalance

If anything, IF will balance your hormones. Doing IF wrong will indeed cause leptin and ghrelin, the main hunger hormones, to go crazy and make people binge. Then they will feel guilty and restrict themselves more. The hormones will get even more imbalanced. This effect can suppress a woman's ovulation and even stop her period. However, a woman who implements IF correctly by keeping herself nourished in her eating windows will not experience this at all.

It Will Destroy Your Metabolism

Your metabolism will run on whatever energy source is easiest. Sugar from food is the easiest, so your body burns that first. With no sugar present, the body turns to burn its own fat cells. Either way, your metabolism works. You cannot destroy it.

Some say that if you fast, you will overeat and then have even more trouble losing weight. This problem is psychological, not physiological. Often people hate restrictive diets so much that they do overeat when they stop dieting, causing them to gain the weight back. Then, they are resistant to new diet approaches and have trouble losing the regained weight. Affecting over 80% of people who have dieted, this problem is pretty common. But if you stick with IF and nourish yourself properly, you won't return to overeating, and you won't have this problem. IF doesn't ruin your metabolism to the point where you can't lose weight again if you do gain any back.

It Causes Stress

Technically, fasting is a period of stress. But as Dr. Fung points out, it is good stress that causes your cells to do their work more efficiently and handle the stress of illness more successfully. Therefore, fasting will not cause extra stress.

The first week or so can be stressful because the approach involves change. Relax a lot and do things you enjoy or find soothing. The stress will pass.

Fasting Can Lead to Overeating

If executed with care, you can avoid the urge to binge eat later. It is true that fasting will make you hungry because of your body's hunger signals. The key here is to keep yourself well-nourished when you do eat. Use bone broth to stave off cravings during fasting periods. Also, avoid going on long fasts when you first start. Don't allow the temptation of food around you or have lots of easy snacks in the house as you fast.

Fasting Causes the Body to Go into Starvation Mode

Starvation mode is a myth that some people believe causes the body to hold onto weight when it perceives that it is not getting sufficient calories. Look at any person who has starved themselves, and you will see rapid, immediate weight loss and wasting. That picture of starvation proves that restricting calories to dangerous levels will not cause weight gain, but rather weight loss. Plus, fasting is not a dangerous caloric restriction or starvation, so it will not cause any unhealthy "mode."

Fasting Causes the Body to Burn Muscle

Because fasting stimulates the production of HGH, it builds muscle rather than destroys it. It only promotes your body to eat fat, not muscle. People tend to start losing muscle mass if they consume too few calories or essentially starve themselves. But they will not lose muscle if they stay nourished and hydrated and eat well between fasting periods.

You Can't Work Out While Fasting

You can absolutely work out while fasting. If you have eaten well during your eating window and have some extra body fat, exercise will only make your body burn more. Be sure to stay hydrated for energy.

Chapter 5. Metabolic Effects of Fasting

As we will see, according to its duration, fasting has different repercussions on the organism.

A fast of a few hours must be considered, it is to be considered physiological; it is, in fact, usual in the life of any healthy person, not to eat food for a few hours (generally 4 or 5 or more if you don't eat any kind of snack) after one of the main meals; fasting following normal night's rest is obviously physiological.

Essentially, fasting can be distinguished according to its duration. In most of the cases, we are considering four phases: post-absorption phase, short-term fasting, medium-fasting, long-term fasting.

The post-absorption phase is the one that occurs once the foods that have been taken in the meal have been completely absorbed by the small intestine (incidentally: the second part of the small intestine is called "fasting"). The phase-in question has a duration of about 4-5 hours after which, in general, other food is taken, consequently interrupting the state of fasting.

During the post-absorption phase there is, in the normal subject, a drop in blood glucose levels (lowering of blood sugar); the body "reacts" to this reduction with a process known as hepatic glycogenolysis (degradation of glycogen molecules until glucose is formed), necessary both for maintaining adequate glycaemic levels and for supplying glucose with the other tissues of the body.

In short-term fasting, quantifiable in one day of abstention from food, the metabolic needs of the body are supported, in addition to liver glycogenolysis, also by the oxidation of triglycerides; the glycogen contained in the liver, in fact, is rather limited and it is, therefore, necessary for the body to resort to fatty acids in order to save glucose (intended primarily for the brain and red blood cells).

The organism then uses a metabolic process known as gluconeogenesis; through this process, glucose is synthesized using non-glycidyl precursors (amino acids, glycerol, lactic acid, pyruvate, etc.).

Gluconeogenesis (also neo glycol genesis) has the primary purpose of contributing to the constant maintenance of the blood glucose concentration.

After 24 hours of fasting, you pass into the medium-fasting phase; during this phase, there is a rather marked accentuation of the progress of the gluconeogenesis process. The amino acids that are exploited for this process are those deriving from the degradation of the proteins contained in the muscle tissues (in the human organism there are no deposits of proteins usable for energy purposes); in fact, we are witnessing what is somewhat defined as "cannibalization of the muscles" with a consequent decrease in muscle mass. The appearance of symptoms such as weakness, fatigue, and apathy are inevitable.

The gluconeogenesis process tends, over time, to lose efficacy, so much so that the supply of glucose to the brain is undersized; therefore, the use of ketone bodies (acetone, vinegar acetate, and 3-B-hydroxybutyrate) becomes necessary; these derive from lipid metabolism; in fact, in the absence of sugars, lipids cannot be used for energy purposes and the organism is forced to transform them into ketone bodies, substances that have certain characteristics that make them similar to sugars, first of all, their remarkable input speed and speed of use.

Ketosis has the positive effect of lengthening the survival of the organism, but the "side effects" are not lacking, just mention the considerable increase in blood acidity and overwork to which two important organs such as kidneys and liver are subjected to dispose of the body's excess ketones.

As fasting persists, the various tissues, to save as much glucose as possible, are always forced to resort increasingly to lipid oxidation.

After the twenty-fourth day of fasting, the last phase of fasting is passed; without an intervention, the subject is destined to die within a noticeably brief time. The organism, in fact, has exploited all the resources that the liver and blood made available to him and the death comes because of breathing difficulties, dehydration, and breakdown of the immune system. As mentioned, a human being can survive about a month of fasting, although cases of longer fasts have been documented.

Therapeutic (intermittent) Fasting

Considering what is reported in the previous paragraphs it is possible to make some considerations on the question of therapeutic fasting, that is, of that fasting which, used for periods and with appropriate frequencies (for this reason it is also called intermittent), can improve our health.

If in the past, fasting was mainly linked to mystical-religious choices, today it is seen primarily as a form of physical purification and elimination of toxins that should have polluted our body following a wrong diet.

Regardless of the fact that often those who speak of fasting can insert an impressive series of scientific cautionaries while explaining the alleged benefits of the operation, it is possible to show how fasting, even occasional, is actually harmful.

In fact, during a calorie reduction, the organism can carry out an adaptation or accommodation process.

With the adaptation, there is a lowering of the basal metabolism in order to preserve the resources, while with the accommodation the resources are used to compensate for the lack of nutrient supply. In general, the organism tends to use adaptation processes that are not destructive (for example, the lean body is not affected).

With fasting, it is very likely that settling processes will occur, especially if it is protracted.

In fact, gluconeogenesis (i.e., the use of lipids and proteins to obtain the glucose necessary to maintain normal blood glucose values; in a sedentary, glycogen stores are in fact exhausted in less than 24 hours) already after a few days produce negative effects: the lean mass is affected to convert proteins into energy (with consequent liver overload) and fats (with a slimming effect) with the consequent accumulation of ketone waste are also used for the same purpose.

In essence, therapeutic fasting instead of purifying the organism, intoxicates it!

Therapeutic Fasting

Depending on its duration, fasting has different repercussions on the organism.

And fast one day?

One day fasting is also not positive. In fact, a sedentary (for an athlete it would be hard to fast and train) who has a calorie requirement of 1,800-1,900 calories spends about 1,400 of them for the basal metabolic rate. This means that in order to live, the organism, whether fasting or not, produces waste. Purification does not depend on fasting, but on the ability to eliminate these wastes; if this ability fails or simply decreases, fasting cannot restore it.

So, one must ask when fasting starts to hurt, be aware that a good one never does. The answer is in the slag amount which the gluconeogenesis process produces, by disassembling the muscles and burning fat in the presence of low or extremely low carbohydrate reserves to have the necessary energy.

Since gluconeogenesis is used to make up for a lack of energy, the damage to fasting depends on the energy spent by the subject: it is one thing to fast while lying in bed and other is to fast while living an active life. Even a day's fast can hurt.

An anecdote: a boy fasted for about 36 hours due to a mild flu syndrome that had affected the gastrointestinal tract. Having recovered from his illness, he thought it well to play an exhausting ball game.

Result: tear to the adductors. Obviously, there is no counter-test, but it is highly likely that the protein catabolism triggered by fasting and physical effort caused the injury.

Fasting According to Alternative Medicine

According to some hygienist currents, fasting would also have a therapeutic function (as we have seen, they call it therapeutic fasting) and even would heal many diseases, including tumors, thanks to a process of cellular autolysis that would cause tissue renewal.

This theory is only an example of how ignorance of the bases of human physiology tends to support imaginative, purely philosophical theories, completely detached from reality. Needless to comment, I can only cite the case of a teammate of mine who, after having embraced alternative theories, veganism, and others as such for years, he was struck at just over 50 years of age by a tumor in his intestine (a disease that can be treated today with timely conventional intervention); he refused all treatment and, until the very end, believed that fasting could save him. Honor to consistency, but perhaps the children and wife would have preferred that he was still alive.

Thinking that fasting can purify is typical to anorexic mentalities who however believe that food or some foods can do a lot of harm. It goes without saying that in a healthy person it is not clear why slag should accumulate (Which? Where? In what quantity?), which would be eliminated by fasting.

Given that it is fasting that intoxicates the body, if a healthy person is not in balance with his own diet (that is, he cannot naturally cut the waste it produces) it simply means that he eats badly.

Chapter 6. Foods and Drinks Suitable for Intermittent Fasting

Intermittent fasting is highly appealing to many due to the permissive nature of the diet, allowing people to eat their favorite foods freely during the eating window. In theory, this principle works with great success.

In practice, however, we want you to avoid the greatest mistake people make, which is none other than drastic overeating. Indeed, this lifestyle was meant to allow individuals to eat as much and whatever they wanted during the eating window, but it simply cannot apply if the interpretations of "whatever" and "as much" are dramatic.

We've talked about how the base of weight loss and weight gain surrounds caloric intake, eating more calories than you consume adding up to weight gain while eating fewer results in weight loss. Intermittent fasting is not a miracle that can change human physiology, and while you can technically eat whatever you want, practically, it is possible to overestimate the power of fasting and end up gaining weight.

This information is largely left out by individuals talking about intermittent fasting, as it goes against the baseline of this diet, but also because these cases are quite rare. Yet rare does not mean inexistent, and we do not want our readers to fall victim of this convenient trap.

Indeed, intermittent fasting does not require you to count calories or macronutrients, but if one happens to consume an entire cake and a bottle of soda during the eating window, they easily exceed their caloric needs. This simply means that while you do not have to go to extreme lengths to lose weight with intermittent fasting, some obviously unhealthy and fattening foods should still be avoided.

A healthy and balanced diet consists of a variety of vegetables, grains, meats, and fruits. Healthy should be your number one priority. If you happen to eat a basic, balanced diet, without much so-called "junk food", sugary drinks, or desserts, this should not be a problem.

You can still have a slice of cake as a dessert, as the fattening element is not the substance, but the quantity. What you must consider throughout your daily diet, but is especially impactful for fasting, is the use of yoghurts.

This being, our first specific food we want to talk about, yoghurts and low-fat, light dairy products, can heavily impact satiation. This trick is oftentimes used by bodybuilders; whose appetites are immensely more demanding. Eating or drinking a glass of yoghurt or sour milk will fulfill your hunger, as it fills your stomach while maintaining a low caloric value.

For fasting, especially with your last meal of the day, you are aiming to be satiated for as long as possible, which makes sour milk and low-fat yoghurts a formidable addition.

The other massive pillar comes under the general name of fresh vegetables. Cucumbers, tomatoes, salad, cabbage, etc. will grant you more satiation for very, very low caloric values. Other than the convenience, we have the added health benefits in the form of essential vitamins which are obtained from such vegetables.

Not only delicious, healthy, and satiating, vegetables also fall into the less expensive category of foods, granting even more convenience, which intermittent fasting relies on.

While sour milk and yoghurts might not be everyone's favorites, vegetables can be prepared and seasoned in such a vast variety of ways that anyone can find an enjoyable form.

Not to be mistaken for foods such as French fries, which take one already more heavily caloric vegetable and add more calories to the mix by deep frying it. Under fresh vegetables we mean either raw or mildly cooked, fulfilling, and low-calorie veggies.

An obvious role in any healthy diet goes to meats. Slightly biased by our love for this type of food, meats are considered a must, but try controlling the way they are cooked. Eating fried chicken once a day will not represent an issue, but only consuming deep-fried meat will.

Protein, the main component in meats, is known for being highly satiating and healthy, making it one of the most important macronutrients, especially for individuals who engage in physical training. It goes without saying that meats do not fall into any negative category, but one part which should be looked upon is the cholesterol content of the specific kind.

For older or obese individuals, the excess of high-cholesterol meats can mean trouble, in which case we recommend fish, low-fat meats, and seafood in terms of meat.

Finally, one more macronutrient worth mentioning in dietary fiber. The key to the relevance of dietary fiber stands in how satiating it is. For everyone who hasn't yet had a bowl of oatmeal, we advise you to give it a try, spiced up with cinnamon, fruits, or even some dark chocolate chips.

I specifically remember eating oatmeal for the first time, and how amazed I was by the fact that it kept me satiated for hours. This is especially important when it comes to your last meal of the day. Fiber-rich food, in combination with a glass of sour milk and a hefty amount of meats and vegetables, ensure that the remaining four hours before sleep pass without cravings.

Dietary fiber is found in foods such as:

- Oatmeal

- Nuts and Seeds

- Broccoli

- Corn

- Carrots

- Whole wheat pasta

- Whole grain bread

- Peas

- Oranges

Some great sources of protein, if we are already on the subject, will be:

- Fish

- Red meat

- Cottage cheese

- Protein shakes

- Eggs

- Seafood

While the subject of pre-prepared protein and supplement shakes is widely debated by so-called experts, common acceptance stands by the use of such products.

Regardless of age group, different brands offer easy to make snack which can act as a complete meal, perfect for intermittent fasting when you time to eat is limited.

A key piece of advice is the use of these products after physical activity or before sleep as a last snack before closing the eating window. What we do have to warn you however is pricing. Certain companies, which we are not going to name but are very well known, promote their supplements extensively with an exaggerated price tag, while the quality is not necessarily better than the one of a regular market product of the same sort. Do your research before actually spending money on supplements, which should apply to all sorts of products, not just protein or dietary shakes.

For individuals with strict medication or supplementation schedules, do NOT miss out on taking your prescription drugs for the sake of intermittent fasting. Those types of supplements or pills rarely have a caloric value, and the risk for reward factor stands strongly on the side of medication.

Do consult with your doctor before doing any major lifestyle changes, especially at a more advanced age, as a medical professional will know better if the changes are suitable for you.

During the fasted period, you can only consume non-caloric drinks, which in a nutshell are black coffee (no sugar, no milk, no creamer), unsweetened tea, and water.

Different brands have been producing zero-calorie versions, or otherwise known as "diet" alternatives, but although usually negligible, a bottle of Coke Zero has about 2 calories. The essence of intermittent fasting consists of consuming 0.

Having covered a general point of view over the foods which are best suited for this diet, we are now going to cover some highly effective tips and tricks to help you through your journey.

Chapter 7. Activating Autophagy

What if there is a way to stay forever young? What if you could erase a couple of years from your face and skin and take off some inches from your waistline by activating an internal cleanup process? Would you not want to know how to do that? Well, staying forever young or finding a literal fountain of youth might be unlikely, but you can stimulate a natural process to keep cells rejuvenated and functioning optimally for the rest of your life. That process is known as autophagy.

What Is Autophagy and How Does It Work?

Reduce, reuse, and recycle is a popular phrase you're likely to hear in discussions relating to environmental sustainability. In many ways, this is similar to autophagy, which means reducing or breaking down and repairing part of the cell, and then recovering important body chemicals that can be reused by the liver.

In a nutshell, autophagy is the natural process that removes toxic materials and broken cells from your body to create new and healthier cells. The term comes from Latin, which translates to self-eating (auto= "self" and phagy= "to eat"). In a weird way, this means your body is eating itself! Don't panic, it's a good thing. It's a rejuvenation process for your body.

If you fully realize what autophagy is and how to make it work for you, you will be quick to find ways to consciously stimulate the process because it can keep you feeling and looking younger than your real age! Older adults, in particular, can use this natural process to increase longevity.

Here's a simple analogy of how autophagy works that I think a lot of women can relate to. Think of what happens inside your kitchen when you are preparing a delicious meal. You are creating something heartfelt and necessary while at the same time making a mess and producing waste. If you leave your kitchen dirty after preparing your meal, it will be difficult to make your next meal. So, you do what any self-respecting woman does: throw or put away leftovers, clean the counter, put away unused ingredients, and recycle some of the food if you can. This is exactly how autophagy works in your body. It cleans up after you!

A big mess is created each day inside the body. This mess includes parts of dead cells, damaged proteins, and harmful particles that prevent optimal body function. When you were much younger, the process of autophagy cleared this mess up as quickly as possible, keeping you looking young and supple. But as you grow older, the cleanup process slows down. Dirt, mess, and crumbs start to build up internally due to old age. If left unattended, the buildup can result in rapid aging, increased risk of cancer and dementia, as well as other diseases associated with old age.

But growing older doesn't mean you're doomed to have an inefficient cellular cleaning process. You can stimulate the process of autophagy and make it work as it used to when you were a lot younger. An effective way to do that is by doing something that induces stress such as decreasing insulin levels and increasing your glucagon levels. In simpler terms, go without food for longer than you usually would. When you get really hungry as you do when you fast, your glucagon is increased and stimulates autophagy.

You can achieve some positive life-altering benefits by simply activating autophagy. But before going into the immense health benefits, let us consider the science behind the process, albeit briefly.

The Science Behind Autophagy

Autophagy in humans is induced by the activation of a protein known as p62. As soon as broken or damaged cells caused by metabolic byproducts begin to appear, p62 stimulates the process of clearing up the clutter on a cellular level. All remaining parts of waste or damaged cells that can lead to health problems are reduced, reused, and recycled. Think of the process as decluttering on a cellular level. The entire process is neatly executed to keep you healthy, strong to handle any biological stress, and of course, keep you looking and feeling young.

Researchers from Newcastle University found that humans evolved to live longer by responding well to biological stressors (Newcastle

University, 2018). Usually, fruit flies can't withstand stress. But when researchers genetically altered fruit flies by giving them the human version of p62, they found that the fruit flies lived longer than usual, even under stressful conditions.

The Benefits

Some people are said to have different biological and chronological ages. That is to say, their age is different from their quality of their life. Women are more likely to worry about showing signs of aging or looking older than men. Thankfully, you can look younger by activating autophagy. What the process does to your cells is to remove toxins and recycle cells instead of creating new ones. These rejuvenated cells will behave like new and work better.

Your skin is constantly exposed to harmful lights, air, chemicals, as well as harsh weather conditions. This causes damage to your skin cells. As the damaged cells continue to accumulate, your skin begins to wrinkle, lose elasticity, and no longer appear smooth. The process of autophagy repairs your skin cells that might have been partly damaged to make your skin glow and healthier. In the same way that wear and tear happen with things you use frequently, wear and tear (microtear) also happen to your muscles as you use them, especially during exercises. Your muscles become inflamed and require repairs. What this means is you need more energy to use these specific muscles. The process of autophagy in your cells will degrade the damaged parts in the muscle, reduce the amount of energy sent to the muscle, and ensure energy balance.

To keep your metabolism working well, your cells need to be in top shape. The powerhouse of your cell is the mitochondria. A lot of harmful trash is left behind in the mitochondria as it performs its function of burning fat and making adenosine triphosphate (ATP) – the molecule that stores all the energy you need to do almost everything. This harmful trash can damage your cells. Autophagy ensures that these toxins are promptly taken care of to prevent damage to your cells and keep them in a healthy state.

Several processes and activities that occur during your cellular cleaning and repairs also help you to maintain a healthy weight. For example, when toxins are removed from your cells through autophagy and you successfully excrete them, your fat cells can no longer store these toxins. Also, when you fast for short periods (12 to 16 hours), autophagy is activated, fat-burning also takes place, and since it is not a prolonged fast, your proteins are spared. All these activities and processes help to make you leaner and fitter.

The cells of your gastrointestinal tract hardly ever take breaks. You put them to work consistently, and this can affect digestive health. Autophagy helps repair and restore the cells. When you stop eating for long periods, you give your gut ample time to rest and heal. Giving your gut some rest (from digesting your meal) is vital for overall improved digestive health.

Certain neurodegenerative diseases, such as Alzheimer's disease and Parkinson's disease, are caused by excessive accumulation of damaged proteins around brain cells. Autophagy clears this clutter of damaged proteins that don't work as they should. Dementia is not a normal part of aging, although it has a lot to do with older people. If your brain cells are clear of clutter (damaged protein cells), you will perform cognitive functions optimally.

How to Activate Autophagy

As already stated, one of the quickest ways to activate autophagy is by staying away from food for longer periods. In other words, intermittent fasting can create just the right level of stress on your body to kick start the internal cleanup process. Going without food leads to an energy deficit, and that induces autophagy ridding your body of decaying cells and accumulated junk. So, besides the widely known weight-loss benefits of intermittent fasting, perhaps a far-reaching positive aspect of practicing intermittent fasting is activating autophagy.

Physical exercise is another stress-inducing activity that can stimulate autophagy. Some of the areas of the body where exercise induces autophagy are the liver, muscles, and pancreas.

When you combine intermittent fasting with moderate physical exercises, you are taking autophagy to a new level.

Chapter 8. Ideal Diet in Menopause

When our bodies begin to change, some essential natural transitions are too often negatively affected. It is imperative to learn how to change our eating habits and eating patterns appropriately. It often happens that a woman is not ready for this new condition and experiences it with a feeling of defeat as an inevitable sign of time travel. This feeling of prostration turns out to be too invasive and involves many aspects of one's stomach.

Therefore, it is necessary to remain calm as soon as there are messages about the first signs of change in our human body, ward off the onset of menopause for the right purpose, and minimize the adverse effects of suffering, especially in the early days. Even during this challenging transition, targeted nutrition can be very beneficial.

What Happens to the Body of a Menopausal Woman?

There are no significant weight fluctuations. It will undoubtedly support women going through menopause, but that it is not a sufficient condition to present with classic symptoms that are felt, which can be classified according to the period experienced. We can distinguish between the pre-menopausal phase, which lasts around 45 to 50 years, and is physiologically compatible with a drastic reduction in the hormone estrogen production (responsible for the menstrual cycle, which starts irregularly.) This period is accompanied by a series of complex and highly subjective endocrine changes. Compare effectively: headache, depression, anxiety, and sleep disorders.

When someone enters actual menopause, estrogen hormone production decreases even more dramatically, the range of the symptoms widens, leading to large amounts of the hormone, for example, to a particular class called catecholamine adrenaline. The result of these changes is a dangerous heat wave, increased sweating, and the presence of tachycardia, which can be more or less severe.

However, the changes also affect the female genital organs, with the volume of the breasts, uterus, and ovaries decreasing. The mucous membranes become less active, and vaginal dryness increases. There may also be changes in bone balance, with decreased calcium intake and increased mobilization at the skeletal system's expense. Thus, there is a lack of continuous bone formation, and conversely, erosion begins, which is a predisposition for osteoporosis.

Although menopause causes significant changes that significantly change a woman's body and soul, metabolism is the worst. In fact, during menopause, the absorption and accumulation of sugars and triglycerides change. It is easy to increase some clinical values such as cholesterol and triglycerides, which lead to high blood pressure arteriosclerosis. Besides, many women often complain of disturbing circulatory disorders and local edema, especially in the stomach. It also makes weight gain more straightforward, even though you haven't changed your eating habits.

The Ideal Diet for Menopause

In cases where disorders related to the arrival of menopause become challenging to manage, drug, or natural therapy under medical supervision may be necessary. The contribution given by a correct diet at this time can be considerable. In fact, given the profound variables that come into play, it is necessary to modify our food routine, both in order not to be surprised by all these changes and to adapt in the most natural way possible.

The drop-in estrogen always causes the problem of fat accumulation in the abdominal area. It is also responsible for most women's classic hourglass shape, which consists of depositing fat mainly on the hips, which begins to fail with menopause. As a result, we go from a gynoid condition to an android one, with a greasy increase localized on the belly. Besides, the metabolic rate of disposal is reduced. Even if you do not change your diet and eat the same quantities of food as you always have, you could experience weight gain, which will be more marked in the presence of bad habits or an irregular diet. The digestion is also slower and intestinal function becomes more complicated. It further contributes to swelling and intolerance and digestive disorders that have never been disturbed before. Therefore, the beginning will be more problematic and challenging to manage during this period. The distribution of nutrients must be different: reducing the amount of low carbohydrate, which is always preferred not to be purified, helps avoid the peak of insulin and at the same time maintains stable blood sugar.

Furthermore, it will be necessary to increase the quantity of both animal and vegetable proteins slightly; choose good fats, prefer seeds and extra virgin olive oil, and severely limit saturated fatty acids (those of animal origin such as lard). All this and the proportion of antioxidants taken will help counteract the effect of free radicals, whose concentration begins to raise during this period.

It is necessary to prefer foods rich in phytoestrogens, which will help control the states of stress the body is subjected. This will favor, at least in part, the overall estrogenic balance.

These molecules are divided into three main groups, and the foods that contain them should never be missing on our tables. They are: a) flavones, present mainly in legumes such as soy and red clover; b) lignans, of which flax seeds and oily seeds in general, are rich; and c) coumestans, found in sunflower seeds, beans, and sprouts. A calcium supplement will be necessary through cheeses such as parmesan; dairy products such as yogurt, egg yolk, some vegetables such as rocket, Brussels sprouts, broccoli, spinach, asparagus; legumes; dried fruit such as nuts, almonds, or dried grapes.

Excellent additional habits that will help to regain well-being may be: limiting sweets to sporadic occasions, thus drastically reducing sugars (for example, by giving up sugar in coffee and getting used to drinking it bitter); learn how to dose alcohol a lot (avoiding spirits, liqueurs, and aperitif drinks) and choose only one glass of good wine when you are in company, this because it tends to increase visceral fat which is what is going to settle at the abdominal level. Even by eating lots of fruit, it isn't easy to reach a high carbohydrate quota as in a traditional diet. However, a dietary plan to follow can be useful for a more precise indication of how to distribute the foods. One's diet must be structured personally, based on specific metabolic needs and one's lifestyle.

Chapter 9. Is Intermittent Fasting Safe for Older Adults?

This transition from glucose to ketones as an energy source also changes healthy body chemistry. When women reach 50, their bodies brace for and progress through menopause and its aging side effects. To maintain their health, many women need to take new and different approaches, including adapting their diets to obtain the required nutrients. They will want to look at the right diets for women over 50, in that case.

Kay also cites osteoporosis, osteoarthritis, and changes in blood sugar regulation (insulin resistance may occur due to changes in hormones), as other conditions women may experience in this age group. Registered dietician Kayla Hulsebus, MS, RD, LD, explains that women can modify their diets to adapt better to their bodies' natural changes. Along this book, we will be sharing tips and advices on Intermittent fasting, or rather, lifestyles that can help support healthy muscle mass, hormone balance and proper weight management for women over 50.

After 50, many women want to lose weight. Unfortunately, with nature playing tricks on their metabolisms, it feels twice as hard to move those pounds. Most have found that green tea, with its many health benefits, does not function. It is not going to shrink one to two sizes of dresses. Life is getting stronger and simpler for all of us, even as we grow older. But unfortunately, some things don't get easier with age, like weight loss. In reality, it can feel harder than ever to drop unwanted pounds. If it's a packed life or sore knees that keep you off, maybe you're less motivated to go to the gym. In your 50s and 60s, those 10 pounds that you gained in your 40s can become an extra 20 pounds. But experts believe that focusing on keeping your healthier weight at any age is vital.

"Excess weight is something we shouldn't disregard no matter how old we are," says Robert Huizenga, MD, a clinical medicine internist and associate professor at UCLA. The good news is that while it is much harder to lose weight in your 50s, women actually won't find it harder to lose weight than men.

What to Consider Before You Start Your Journey to Weight Loss

For example, talking to the doctor before initiating some new fitness routine is more important than ever. "Medical issues, such as heart disease and metabolic disease, become more common after age 60, so it is much more important to have a medical check-up before attempting a fat loss plan," Dr. Huizenga commented. The fact is that your oxygen intake can be reduced by up to one-third of what it was at 25. This could make it harder to take deep breaths while you are doing exercise. That is why easing into a new workout regimen is key. This is also a decade when your hips, knees, and other key joints are more likely to develop arthritis, which means you may need to switch from running or aerobic exercise to swimming and/or a gentle walking plan.

5 Tips for Intermittent Fasting Everyone Should Know

It has been done for decades now, and honestly, I can remember when I started fasting for the first time. Back in the early 1990s, fasting was just what strange health freaks would do. Very few people can understand fasting, let alone choose to take part in it. Now we've finished the work, completed hundreds, if not thousands, of experiments, and the conclusion is unanimous: Intermittent Fasting works!

Before Intermittent Fasting, here are 5 of my top secrets I think everyone should consider:

Prepare to Your Fast

Preparation is a good idea, as simple as replacing three meals with a milkshake. This will reduce your calorie intake and increase your nutrient intake before the day you plan to fast. This makes your system ready and reduces the greatest amount of physical and mental discomfort that could come with fasting.

Use Supplements to Make Your Fasting Days Better

You can use specially formulated supplements instead of only doing regular water fasts that will significantly boost the performance during a quick. The supplements work like inputting a programming code into a machine. You're putting in the code, and the code tells the computer what to do and supports it in doing the job it's told to.

It Might Not Be Any More

First, do single-day cleanses, then split cleanses over two days. A single day of cleansing or fasting is quite powerful, and on day 2, you will experience 80 percent more fat burning when you do a second in a row.

On Fasting Days, Drink More Tea

Water works as a vehicle for carrying nutrients through your body and helps eliminate them. Generally, if you sweat, exercise, or use your body more than average, it is between 2 and 3 liters per day, or even more.

Make Fasting Days More Like Days of Rest

Keeping your workout to a minimum and not overdoing it may help you clean up better. Your body can only do one thing at a time, so you can either exercise or cleanse yourself. Decide what you're doing, focus, and do just that.

Common Mistakes to Avoid During Intermittent Fasting

Mistake 1: You Can Only Drink Water in the Fasted State

Although this being really successful, it's not the only way to do it. In the fasted state, getting green tea may be helpful to you. Studies have found green tea is encouraging weight loss. Black coffee is great for those who love coffee in its fasted state. You can also make bulletproof coffee after a ketogenic diet, but if you eat carbs, try avoiding the coffee because it does more harm than good in losing fat and calories.

Mistake 2: Being Overly Ambitious with Fasting

You had your body when you started with intermittent fasting at first. Instead of thinking that you can change your lifelong eating habit overnight, you can go ahead and eat a few hours into it if you crave food. It takes your body a few weeks to get used to the fasting, but make sure you drive those cheaters farther away before you hit the point where you can forget about the food, and when you start, you wouldn't want to look back.

Mistake 3: The Longer Your Fast, the Better

That is not the case. Fasting benefits tend to go down after 20-24 hours. However, some studies recommend achieving more benefits when we fast for 24 hours, but it needs to be done once a week.

Therefore, starvation mode comes into play within 72-96 hours without food that is about 3-4 days. So please keep it simple and do not go overboard with a fast time.

Mistake 4: The Feeling of Hunger Is Bad for You

"It's too late when you're hungry" This is full bullshit and pure science. Intermittent fasting will make your muscle lean without too much fat, so don't feel hungry until you feel hungry. At one point, everybody feels hungry, so the feeling is just natural; just embrace it. The more you get used to fasting, though, the less hungry you'll get.

Mistake 5: Intermittent Fasting Is Not Good for Our Health

This is another old saying that sticks with no evidence if it is true or not. Intermittent fasting is, in fact, one of the highly effective methods available as a last resort for burning fats as energy. Your body is depleted in the fasted state of glycogen and blood glucose so that the body is forced to use fats as energy. The body is ready to enter the fasted state when you wake up and fast for like 8 hours. Typically, when we break the fast and have what is called "Breakfast," that's what I describe as the day's first mistake. Continue to fly a few more hours and work out before eating your first meal to reap its daytime benefits.

Mistake 6: Not Taking Enough Minerals

Elements like calcium, magnesium, and potassium when you're fasting are so important. Minerals don't affect your metabolism concerning calories in and out. Minerals are so important to cellular processes, and our brain sends out electrical signals in our whole body. The brain can't function well if you don't have them, so you can add the minerals to your water jug and drink it when you're fasting.

Mistake 7: Consuming Branched Chain Amino Acids

Yeah! Some studies were conducted on the topic. A group of 5 men was selected, and their levels of energy substrate, amino acids, and insulin were checked during their fast. They took their baseline blood sample on day 1 and then began fasting. 5 days later, at the beginning of their fast, 5 grams of branched-chain amino acids were given. The results showed they had a small spike of insulin throughout the day (note that a small spike of insulin in the body makes fasting over as you can't get into ketosis).

Mistake 8: Not Exercising

One of the strangest things some people say that there's no science to break it down is that you shouldn't do any exercise while you're fasting. This is absolutely not true! Exercising helps activate the metabolism when fasting. You are in the sympathetic mode of the nervous system when you are in a state of fasting. If you're doing an intense workout, you'll trigger the sympathetic nervous system that starts oxidation and lipolysis (the lipid breakdown) involving triglyceride hydrolysis into glycerol and free fatty acids, which means that fats are mobilized. So, you'll definitely get double mobilization when you double it up. In fact, the human growth hormone rises enormously when you're eating and exercising, which consequently increases the degradation and accumulation of fatty acids.

I hope we managed to clear up certain myths about intermittent fasting. When you really get into that habit, it'll feel natural, so you'll give it a trial and reap many rewards.

Sample Daily Plan for Intermittent Fasting

Now that you have learned how to use intermittent fasting to lose fat, let's see how it looks to someone who needs to eat 2,000 calories to lose fat in a real-life setting:

- 7:00 am Wake. Drink a big glass of water and some black coffee.

- 10:00 am: Drink some sparkling water for appetite suppression.

- 12:00 pm-1 pm: Meal with calories. (Example: grilled chicken sandwich, French fries, grilled vegetables, and Greek yogurt strawberry.)

- 5:00 pm: A black coffee and a mild apple.

- 6:00 pm: 40-minute full-body exercise lifting weight.

- 6:45 pm: Drink protein shake from the whey and take a shower.

- 7.30pm-8:00pm: Calorie meal 700. (For example, steaks, roasted potatoes, beans, and asparagus)

- 9:00 pm: Decaf green tea.

- 11:00 pm: Sleep

Chapter 10. The Right Mindset When Starting IF

When setting out on your intermittent fasting journey, it's important to keep in mind that success is built on several good practices.

The best part is that these secrets are really easy to implement into your routine. So, don't be afraid to give them a try.

The Difference Between Needing and Wanting to Eat

It is of the utmost importance for you to recognize when you are really hungry and when you think you are hungry.

There Is a Huge Difference Here

If you are guilty of this, it's time that you started noticing what triggers these cravings. For instance, if you overeat when you are anxious, then it might be a good idea for you to pay close attention to these instances. That can make a significant difference in your overall success.

Eat Only When Needed

When you are able to recognize when you eat without being hungry, you begin to create a discipline in which you eat only when needed.

The easiest way to do this is to build a schedule and then stick to it. Building a rather strict schedule will help you accustom your body to eating only when really needed.

Hydration Is Essential

Throughout this book, we've talked about how essential it is to hydrate during fast days. While plain water is perfectly healthy, it should also be mentioned that fruit and vegetable juices are a great source of nutrition.

Ideally, you would consume these juices without any added sugar. Generally speaking, most fruits and vegetables have very few calories. So, you won't blow your calorie budget during fast days. Moreover, most fruits don't have a high glucose content. For instance, apples and lemons don't have much glucose. However, oranges and bananas do. Thus, you want to stick to apple juice and lemon water while cutting down a bit of orange juice. If you can get fresh oranges and squeeze them, you could build a winning formula without consuming needless sugar.

Take Things Slowly

To make this easier, you could use the following rule of thumb. If you are planning to fast on a Monday, you could ramp down your meals, starting with Sunday's lunch. For example, a wholesome lunch (not overdoing it) followed by a very light dinner roughly two hours before bedtime will help you set yourself up for success. Then, consume plenty of water upon getting up on Monday morning. This will keep you full throughout the early morning. Next, make a plan to consume some fruit or non-fat, unsweetened yogurt. This should give you the caloric intake you need. Assuming you are doing a 12-hour fast, plan to have a very light lunch. That way, you won't be burdening your digestive system following the fast. Lastly, you can have a normal dinner, but without overdoing it. The next day, you can go about your usual eating habits.

With this approach, you will never go wrong. You will always feel comfortable at all times during your fasting days.

Cut Down on Carbs and Sugar Even on Non-Fast Days

During non-fast days, you are free to have your usual eating regimen. In fact, folks who try to fast while seriously hooked on sugar and carbs often feel anxious and edgy. They even suffer from mild to serious withdrawal symptoms.

So, the best way to go about it is to cut down on your sugar intake well before attempting to go on a full fast. For instance, you can cut down on your portion sizes roughly two weeks before attempting to do your first fast. That way, you can begin the detoxing process while avoiding any nasty withdrawal symptoms.

Keep Track of Your Achievements

We're going old school here. There is something about writing things down on paper that makes it highly personal. When you do this, you can see how you have been progressing. Make sure to write down the date and the length of each fast. Also, include some notes about the things that went right and the things that didn't go right. That way, you can see how your intermittent fasting regimen has been affecting you both positively and negatively.

Over time, you can look back to see the progress you've made. That's why journaling can be one of the most important things you can do to give yourself the boost you need, especially when you're feeling depressed. We don't recommend using note-taking or journaling apps on your phone or tablet, as they tend to be quite impersonal. Also, a notebook or journal is a very personal item. Please note that this is a very personal journey. As a result, chronicling your accomplishments will allow you to keep things closer to your heart.

CPSIA information can be obtained
at www.ICGtesting.com
Printed in the USA
BVHW090333040521
606332BV00006B/1062